Plant-Based Snacks for Busy People

Quick and Tasty Snacks to Boost Your Plant-Based Diet and Stay Fit

Clay Palmer

Table of Contents

Cumin Olives Snack

Preparation time: 10 minutes Cooking time: 15 minutes
Servings: 4

Ingredients:

1 cup black olives, pitted 1 cup kalamata olives, pitted ½
cup cashew cheese, shredded 2 tablespoons avocado oil
Salt and black pepper to the taste 2 tablespoons cumin,
ground

Directions:

In a bowl, combine the olives with the oil, cashew cheese
and the other ingredients, toss well, spread them on a
baking sheet lined with parchment paper and cook at 390
degrees F for 15 minutes. Divide the olives into bowls
and serve as a snack.

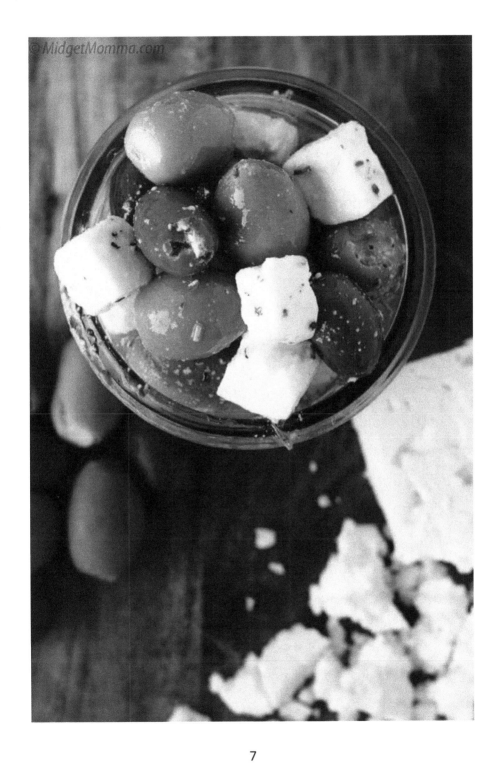

Risotto Bites

Preparation Time: 15 minutes cooking time: 20 minutes serves: 12 bites

Ingredients

½ cup panko bread crumbs 1 teaspoon paprika 1 teaspoon chipotle powder or ground cayenne pepper 1½ cups cold Green Pea Risotto Nonstick cooking spray

Directions

Preparing the Ingredients. Preheat the oven to 425ºF. Line a baking sheet with parchment paper. On a large plate, combine the panko, paprika, and chipotle powder. Set aside. Roll 2 tablespoons of the risotto into a ball. Gently roll in the breadcrumbs, and place on the prepared baking sheet. Repeat to make a total of 12 balls. Spritz the tops of the risotto bites with nonstick cooking spray and bake for 15 to 20 minutes, until they begin to brown. Cool completely before storing in a large airtight container in a single layer (add a piece of parchment paper for a second layer) or in a plastic freezer bag.

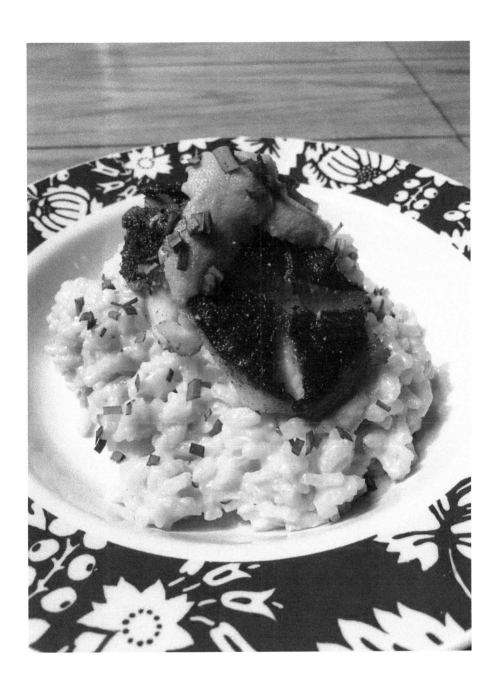

Curried Tofu "Egg Salad" Pitas

Preparation Time: 15 minutes cooking time: 0 minutes serves: 4 sandwiches

Ingredients

1 pound extra-firm tofu, drained and patted dry 1/2 cup vegan mayonnaise, homemade or store-bought 1/4 cup chopped mango chutney, homemade or store-bought 2 teaspoons Dijon mustard 1 tablespoon hot or mild curry powder 1 teaspoon salt 1/8 teaspoon ground cayenne ¾ cup shredded carrots 2 celery ribs, minced 1/4 cup minced red onion 8 small Boston or other soft lettuce leaves 4 (7-inch) whole wheat pita breads, halved

Directions

Crumble the tofu and place it in a large bowl. Add the mayonnaise, chutney, mustard, curry powder, salt, and cayenne, and stir well until thoroughly mixed. Add the carrots, celery, and onion and stir to combine. Refrigerate for 30 minutes to allow the flavors to blend. Tuck a lettuce leaf inside each pita pocket, spoon some tofu mixture on top of the lettuce, and serve.

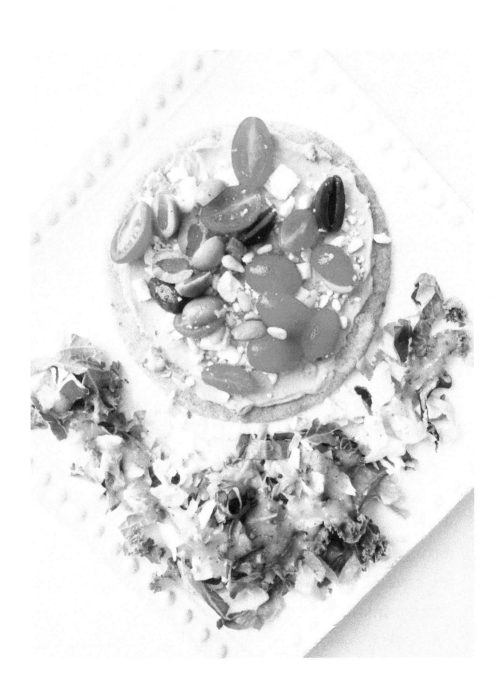

Avocado Cheese Sticks

Preparation time: 15 minutes Cooking time: 25 minutes Servings: 5

Ingredients:

1 large egg 1 large avocado, flesh scooped out, sliced thickly ¼ cup Parmesan cheese ¼ teaspoon garlic powder ¼ teaspoon onion powder ¼ cup organic pork rinds 1 ½ tablespoons heavy cream Pinch of salt Pinch of ground black pepper Olive oil

Directions:

Whisk the egg and heavy cram in a mixing bowl. Continue stirring until smooth and creamy. Set aside. On another bowl, combine Parmesan cheese, garlic powder, onion powder, and pork rinds. Season with salt and pepper. Set aside. Season avocado slices with salt. Coat with egg and cream mixture. Dredge in pork rind mixture. Repeat with the remaining slices. In a pan, heat the olive oil. Once hot, fry the each avocado stick for 1 minute. Immediately remove and drain on paper towels. Let cooked avocado sticks stand for 3 minutes before serving.

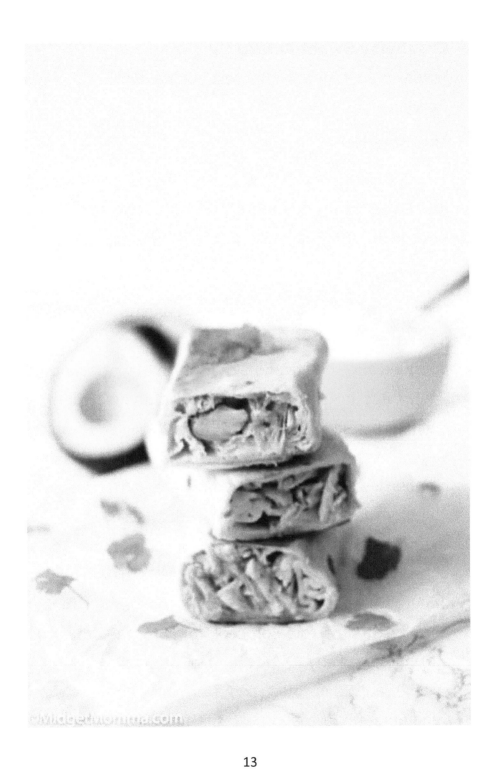

Cranberry Sweet Potato Quiche

Preparation time: 5 minutesCooking time: 45 minutes
Servings: 2

Ingredients:

1 recipe Basic Short-Crust Pastry 2 sweet potatoes 3 ½
lb. carrots ½ lb. cranberries ⅔ cup sugar ½ cup milk 4
eggs ½ lb. soft cream cheese dash of nutmeg dash of salt

Directions:

Prepare the short crust, line an 11-inch quiche pan with
it, and prebake according to Directions. Peel the sweet
potatoes and carrots and either grate them or chop them
finély. Put the vegetables in a pot, douse them with
boiling, salted water, bring to a boil, and cook the
vegetables 5 minutes, then drain them. Wash the
cranberries and pick out any that are soft or blemished.
Put them in an enameled pot with the sugar and cook
them, covered, over low heat for 10 minutes, stirring
occasionally. Remove the lid and cook the berries for 5
minutes more, stirring almost constantly. Add the
potatoes and carrots and cook for 3 to 4 minutes more,
stirring constantly. Beat together the milk, eggs, cream
cheese, a little nutmeg, and a tiny bit of salt. Stir in the
vegetable mixture and pour the filling carefully into the

prepared shell. Bake the quiche in a preheated oven at 375 degrees for 40 minutes, or until the top is golden and the filling firm.

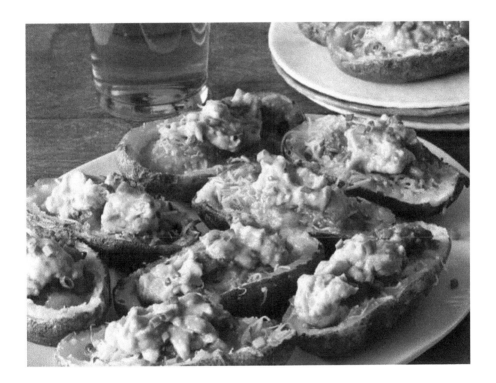

Crepes with Feta Cheese

Preparation time: 5 minutesCooking time: 20 minutes Servings: 2

Ingredients:

3 Tbs. olive oil 1 cup feta cheese, crumbled 2 eggs, lightly beaten 2 cups, farmer cheese, crumbled ½ tsp. dried oregano, crushed ½ tsp. dried dill weed, crushed 2 cloves garlic, minced or crushed fresh-ground black pepper to taste 12 crepes butter for the pan Garnish wedges of cantaloupe

Directions:

Mash the cheeses with a fork until there are no large lumps left. Stir in the olive oil, eggs, and seasonings, combining everything thoroughly. Do not add salt, as the feta cheese is already very salty. Spread a heaping teaspoonful of the filling evenly on ½ of a crepe and fold the other half over it. Now take a slightly rounded teaspoonful of filling and again spread it on ½ the surface of the folded crepe. Fold the crepe over this second layer of filling, so that it is folded in quarters, layered with cheese. Fill all 12 crepes in this manner. Just before serving, sauté the folded crêpes in butter, for several minutes on each side. They should be lightly browned and hot through. Garnish each serving with a wedge of cantaloupe.

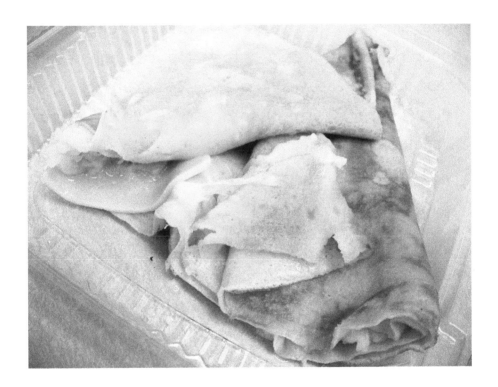

Brie Croquettes

Preparation time: 5 minutesCooking time: 60 minutes
Servings: 2

Ingredients:

1½ cups milk ½ cup flour ½ cup flour 3 eggs, beaten 3 Tbs. olive oil 2 egg yolks 8 oz. Brie, without rind 4 oz. hoop or farmer cheese ⅛ to ¼ tsp. cayenne pepper ¼ tsp. paprika dash of nutmeg ¼ tsp. salt fresh-ground black pepper to taste 1½ to 2 cups fine, dry bread crumbs vegetable oil for deep frying

Directions:

Beat together the flour and milk until the mixture is smooth. Heat it in a medium-sized, heavy-bottomed saucepan, stirring all the while with a whisk until it thickens. As the mixture thickens, beat vigorously to work out lumps. Remove from the heat and whisk in the oil and the egg yolks. Mash the Brie with a wooden spoon until it is a smooth paste, put the hoop cheese through a sieve, and stir the cheeses into the white sauce. Heat the sauce gently, stirring constantly, until the cheeses are melted. Stir in the cayenne, paprika, nutmeg, salt, and pepper. Spread the mixture out evenly on a large plate and chill it until it is firm. Scoop up about 1 tablespoonful of the mixture at a time and drop it into a bowl of flour. Shape it into a round or oval croquette, dip it in the beaten egg, then roll it in the breadcrumbs until it is evenly coated. Continue until the cheese mixture is entirely used up, then start over and dip each croquette again into the beaten eggs and roll it again in the breadcrumbs. It is important to have a solid and even coating of breadcrumbs, or the croquettes will leak when fried. Fry the croquettes in hot oil for only a few minutes. Do as many at one time as will fit in the pot without crowding. They should be golden brown in color. Drain them on paper towels and serve immediately with seasoned rice, on a bed of cooked vegetables, or with a light sauce.

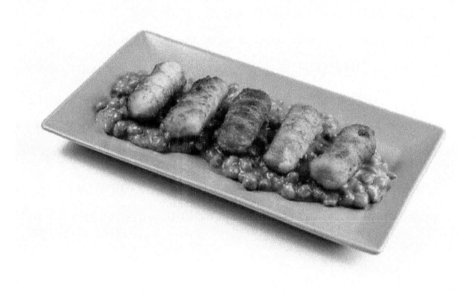

Raw sweet potato pie

Preparation time: 20 minutes | Cooking time: 55 minutes | Servings: 8

Ingredients:

For whole wheat pie crust: ½ cup of coconut oil ½ tsp sea salt 1 ¼ cup whole wheat flour ½ tsp coconut sugar 6-8 tbsp. ice water

For sweet potato filling: 2 ½ cup mashed sweet potatoes ½ cup maple syrup 2 eggs 1 cup almond milk ¼ cup of coconut oil 2 tbsp. whole wheat flour 1 tsp vanilla extract ½ tsp cinnamon ¼ tsp nutmeg ¼ tsp sea salt 2 tbsp. raw pecans Coconut whipped cream: 13.5 oz. coconut milk 1 tbsp. maple syrup ½ tsp vanilla extract

Directions:

Take melted coconut oil, spread it off the parchment paper and freeze it for 15 minutes. Take a blender, add flour, sea salt and coconut sugar and mix well. Add the coconut oil into the mixture and blend until smooth. While blending add 1 tsp ice-cold water until the dough formed. Remove the dough from the blender and wrap it into the paper and put it in the refrigerator for 10 minutes. Take the dough out and unwrap on a clean surface. Rolled the dough well in a round shape and put it into a pie pan or press edge with thumb or folk. Sweet potato filling: Take a large bowl, add mashed potatoes, eggs, maple syrup, coconut oil, vanilla extract, whole wheat flour, almond milk, cinnamon, nutmeg and sea salt. Combine all the Ingredients well. Now put the filling on the whole wheat pie dough and spread evenly. Set the oven on 350 degrees before making potato filling. Put the pie into the oven and bake for 40 to 45 minutes until golden brown. In another bowl, adds maple syrup, coconut milk and vanilla extract and blend them well until frothy. Garnish the potato pie with the coconut cream and serve.

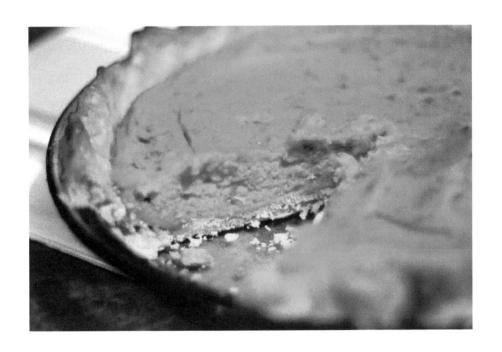

Vegetarian Tacos

Preparation time: 15 minutes Cooking time: 45 minutes
Servings: 5

Ingredients:

1 cup taco sauce 16 oz can vegetarian refried beans,
warmed 1 tsp envelop taco seasoning 2 medium green
peppers cut into half inch slices 12 taco shells, warmed 3
tbsp olive oil 2 medium onions cut into half inch wedges
6 plum tomatoes, seeded and cut into wedges

Directions:

Mix the green peppers, taco seasoning, tomatoes and
onion in a large mixing bowl. Add the oil and toss to
combine. Spread the mixture in a single layer of two
baking pans. Bake uncovered for 20-25 minutes at 475
degrees until it is golden brown. Spread the beans on top
of the taco shells. Scoop the vegetable mixture and
drizzle it with the sauce.

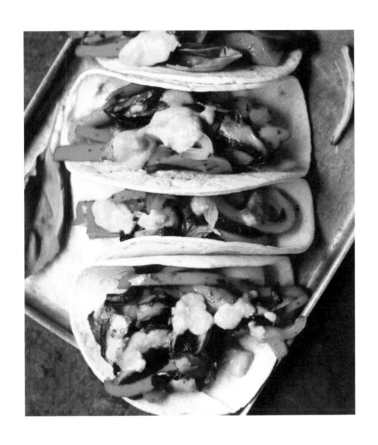

Smoky little devils

Preparation time: 10 minutes | Cooking time: 20 minutes | Servings: 24 pieces

Ingredients:

For hummus: 15oz chickpeas 2 tbsp. lemon juice 2 garlic cloves 1 ½ tbsp. brown mustard Black pepper to taste ¼ tsp salt 1 cup green onion 2 tsp Dijon mustard 1 lemon zest 1 ½ tbsp. lemon juice ½ tsp turmeric For devils: 12 small red potatoes Smoked paprika a pinch 1 green onion Hummus

Directions: For Hummus: In a food processor, add chickpeas, garlic, lemon juice, mustard, pepper, salt and 2 tbsp. water, blend the material until it turns smooth. Now take a small bowl and pour the blended mixture, now add green onion, Dijon mustard, lemon zest, lemon juice and turmeric. Mix all the Ingredients well until combined. Your hummus is ready to use. For devils: Now take a pan full of water and let it boil. When water turns boiling, put the potatoes on a streamer and let them steam for 20 minutes until cooked. Now remove them and let cool. Cut the potatoes from the center and hole their center with a spoon. Now fill each of potato hole with the hummus and sprinkle paprika or green onion for garnishing. Serve the delicious little smoky devils.

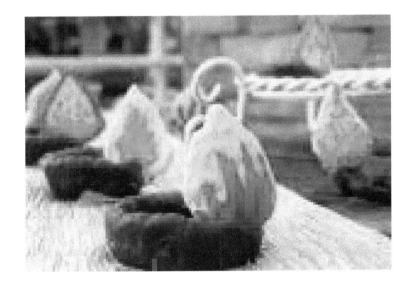

Herb-crusted asparagus spears

Preparation time: 15 minutes | Cooking time: 25 minutes | Servings: 4

Ingredients:

1 bunch of asparagus 1 tsp garlic powder 2 tbsp. hemp seeds 3 garlic cloves ¼ cup yeast 1/8 tsp pepper Paprika a pinch ¼ cup bread crumbs ½ lemon juice

Directions: Wash the bunch of asparagus and let it dry. Cut the bunch from the bottom and separate each of them. Now take a bowl pour hemp seeds, add yeast, garlic powder, minced garlic cloves, paprika and breadcrumbs. Mix them well until combined and set aside. Preheat oven at 350 degrees. Take a baking dish and set asparagus by coating with the hemp mixture. Bake the asparagus for 20 to 25 minutes until crispy. Sprinkle some lemon juice and serve.

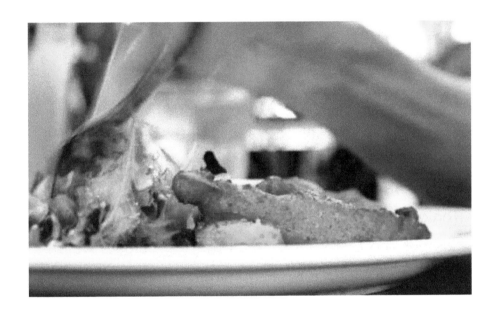

Pea guacamole

Preparation time: 5 minutes | Cooking time: 30 minutes | Servings: 2

Ingredients:

2 cup of frozen green peas ½ tsp cumin 1 tsp garlic crushed 1 tomato chopped ¼ cup fresh lime juice 4 onion chopped ½ cup cilantro chopped ½ tsp hot sauce Sea salt

Directions:

Take a blender and add peas, garlic, lime juice and cumin. Blend all Ingredients well until they turn smooth. Pour the mixture into a small bowl. Add tomato, green onion, cilantro and hot sauce with the mixture. Add salt as per the taste and mix all the Ingredients well. Put it into the refrigerator for 30 minutes and serve.

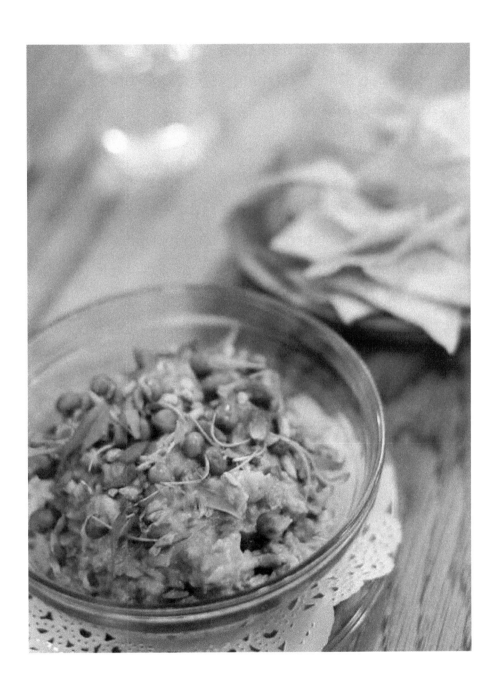

Avocado And Tempeh Bacon Wraps

Preparation Time: 10 minutes cooking time: 8 minutes serves: 4 wraps

Ingredients

2 tablespoons olive oil 8 ounces tempeh bacon, homemade or store-bought 4 (10-inch) soft flour tortillas or lavash flat bread 1/4 cup vegan mayonnaise, homemade or store-bought 4 large lettuce leaves 2 ripe Hass avocados, pitted, peeled, and cut into 1/4-inch slices 1 large ripe tomato, cut into 1/4-inch slices

Directions

In a large skillet, heat the oil over medium heat. Add the tempeh bacon and cook until browned on both sides, about 8 minutes. Remove from the heat and set aside. Place 1 tortilla on a work surface. Spread with some of the mayonnaise and one-fourth of the lettuce and tomatoes. Pit, peel, and thinly slice the avocado and place the slices on top of the tomato. Add the reserved tempeh bacon and roll up tightly. Repeat with remaining Ingredients and serve.

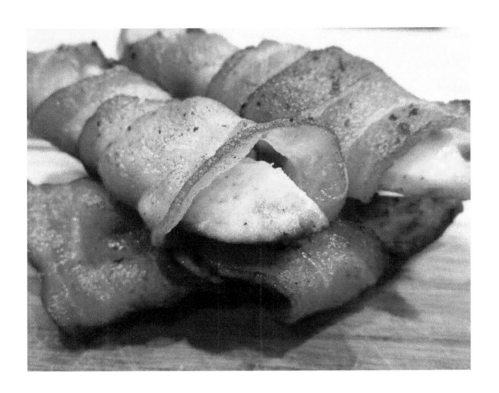

Savory Roasted Chickpeas

Preparation Time: 5 minutes cooking time: 25 minutes serves: 1 cup

Ingredients

1 (14-ounce) can chickpeas, rinsed and drained, or 1½ cups cooked 2 tablespoons tamari, or soy sauce 1 tablespoon nutritional yeast 1 teaspoon smoked paprika, or regular paprika 1 teaspoon onion powder ½ teaspoon garlic powder

Directions

Preparing the Ingredients. Preheat the oven to 400°F. Toss the chickpeas with all the other ingredients and spread them out on a baking sheet. Bake for 20 to 25 minutes, tossing halfway through. Bake these at a lower temperature, until fully dried and crispy, if you want to keep them longer. You can easily double the batch, and if you dry them out they will keep about a week in an airtight container.

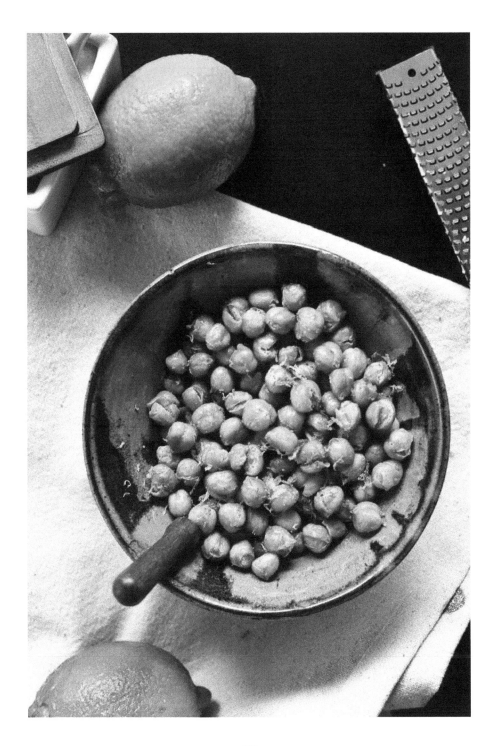

Tomato and Basil Bruschetta

Preparation Time: 10 minutes cooking time: 6 minutes serves: 12 bruschetta

Ingredients

3 tomatoes, chopped ¼ cup chopped fresh basil 1 tablespoon olive oil pinch of sea salt 1 baguette, cut into 12 slices 1 garlic clove, sliced in half

Directions

Preparing the Ingredients. In a small bowl, combine the tomatoes, basil, olive oil, and salt and stir to mix. Set aside. Preheat the oven to 425°F. Place the baguette slices in a single layer on a baking sheet and toast in the oven until brown, about 6 minutes. Flip the bread slices over once during cooking. Remove from the oven and rub the bread on both sides with the sliced clove of garlic. Top with the tomato-basil mixture and serve immediately.

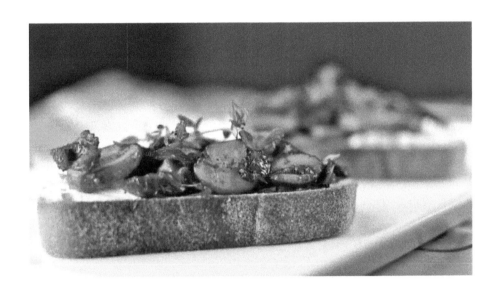

Tempeh Tantrum Burgers

Preparation Time: 15 minutes cooking time: 0 minutes serves: 4 burgers

Ingredients

8 ounces tempeh, cut into 1/2-inch dice ¾ cup chopped onion 2 garlic cloves, chopped ¾ cup chopped walnuts 1/2 cup old-fashioned or quick-cooking oats 1 tablespoon minced fresh parsley 1/2 teaspoon dried oregano 1/2 teaspoon dried thyme 1/2 teaspoon salt 1/4 teaspoon freshly ground black pepper 3 tablespoons olive oil Dijon mustard 4 whole grain burger rolls Sliced red onion, tomato, lettuce, and avocado

Directions:

In a medium saucepan of simmering water, cook the tempeh for 30 minutes. Drain and set aside to cool. In a food processor, combine the onion and garlic and process until minced. Add the cooled tempeh, the walnuts, oats, parsley, oregano, thyme, salt, and pepper. Process until well blended. Shape the mixture into 4 equal patties. In a large skillet, heat the oil over medium heat. Add the burgers and cook until cooked thoroughly and browned on both sides, about 7 minutes per side. Spread desired amount of mustard onto each half of the rolls and layer each roll with lettuce, tomato, red onion, and avocado, as desired. Serve immediately.

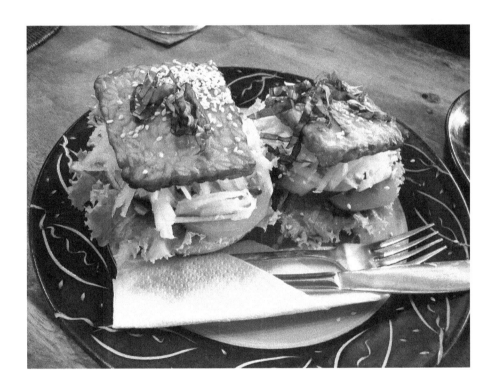

Mushroom Bites

Preparation time: 10 minutes Cooking time: 20 minutes Servings: 4

Ingredients:

1 pound baby Bella mushroom caps 1 teaspoon garlic powder 2 tablespoons olive oil Salt and black pepper to the taste 1 teaspoon curry powder 1 tablespoon parsley, chopped

Directions: In a bowl, mix the mushrooms with the oil, garlic powder and the other ingredients and toss well. Spread the mushrooms on a baking sheet lined with parchment paper and cook in the oven at 350 degrees F for 20 minutes. Arrange on a platter and serve as an appetizer.

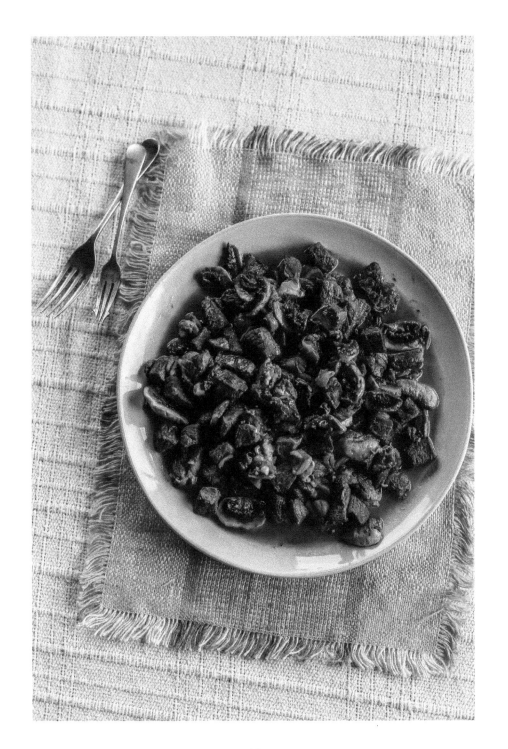

Zucchini Balls

Preparation time: 10 minutes Cooking time: 8 minutes Servings: 6

Ingredients:

2 tablespoons flaxseed mixed with 3 tablespoons water 1 pound zucchinis, grated Salt and black pepper to the taste ¼ cup almond flour 1 cup cilantro, chopped ½ teaspoon garlic powder 2 tablespoons sun dried tomatoes, chopped 2 tablespoons olive oil

Directions: In a bowl, mix the zucchinis with the flaxseed and the other ingredients except the oil, stir well and shape medium balls out of this mix. Heat up a pan with the oil over medium high heat, drop the balls, cook them for 4 minutes on each side, drain excess grease on paper towels, arrange them on a platter and serve.

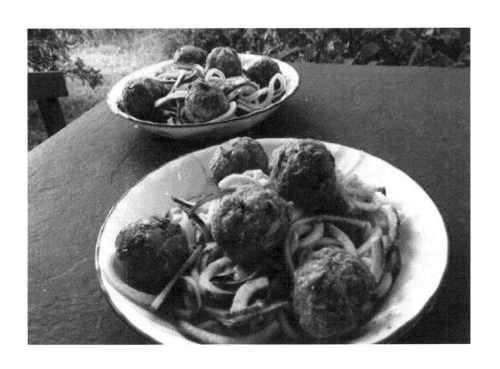

Ultimate Mulled Wine

Servings: 6 Preparation time: 35 minutes

Ingredients:

1 cup of cranberries, fresh 2 oranges, juiced 1 tablespoon of whole cloves 2 cinnamon sticks, each about 3 inches long 1 tablespoon of star anise 1/3 cup of honey 8 fluid ounce of apple cider 8 fluid ounce of cranberry juice 24 fluid ounce of red wine

Directions:

Using a 4 quarts slow cooker, add all the ingredients and stir properly. Cover it with the lid, then plug in the slow cooker and cook it for 30 minutes on thee high heat setting or until it gets warm thoroughly. When done, strain the wine and serve right away

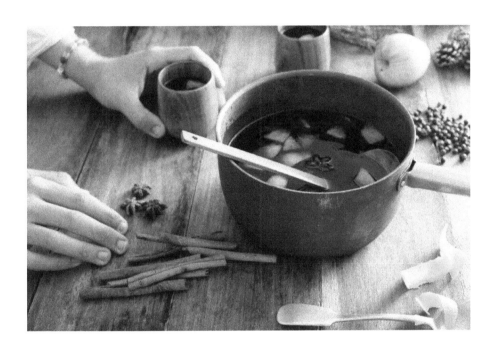

Pineapple, Banana & Spinach Smoothie

Preparation Time: 10 minutes Cooking Time: 0 minute Servings: 1

Ingredients:

½ cup almond milk ¼ cup yogurt 1 cup spinach 1 cup banana 1 cup pineapple chunks 1 tbsp. chia seeds

Direction:

Add all the ingredients in a blender. Blend until smooth. Chill in the refrigerator before serving.

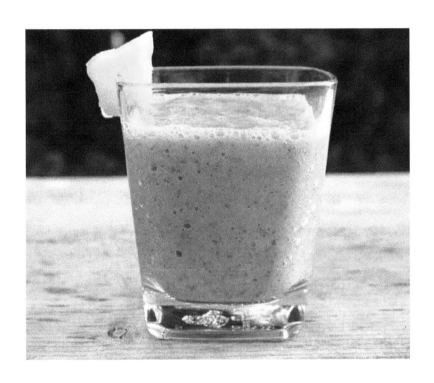

Tart Raspberry Crumble Bar

Preparation time: 10 minutesCooking time: 55 minutes

Servings: 9

Ingredients:

1/2 cup whole toasted almonds 1 cup almond flour 1 cup cold, unsalted butter, cut into cubes 2 eggs, beaten 3-ounce dried raspberries What you'll need from the store cupboard: 1/4 teaspoon salt 3 tbsp MCT or coconut oil.

Directions

In a food processor, pulse almonds until chopped coarsely. Transfer to a bowl. Add almond flour and salt into the food processor and pulse until a bit combined. Add butter, eggs, and MCT oil. Pulse until you have a coarse batter. Evenly divide batter into two bowls. In the first bowl of batter, knead well until it forms a ball. Wrap in cling wrap, flatten a bit and chill for an hour for easy handling. In the second bowl of batter, add the raspberries. In a pinching motion, pinch batter to form clusters of streusel. Set aside. When ready to bake, preheat oven to 375oF and lightly grease an 8x8-inch baking pan with cooking spray. Discard cling wrap and evenly press dough on the bottom of the pan, up to 1-inch up the sides of the pan, making sure that everything is covered in dough. Top with streusel. Pop in the oven and bake until golden brown and berries are bubbly around 45 minutes. Remove from oven and cool for 20 minutes before slicing into 9 equal bars. Serve and enjoy or store in a lidded container for 10-days in the fridge.

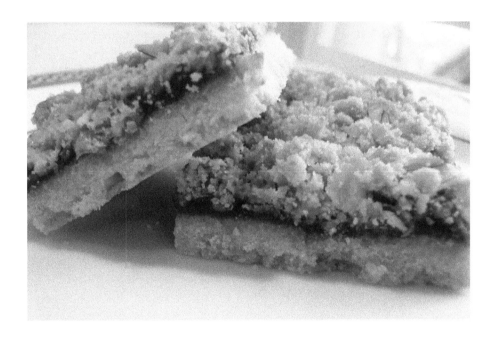

Chives Fennel Salsa

Preparation time: 10 minutes Cooking time: 0 minutes
Servings: 4

Ingredients:

2 fennel bulbs, shredded ½ cup chives, chopped Juice of
1 lime 2 tablespoons olive oil 1 cup black olives, pitted
and sliced Salt and black pepper to the taste 2 celery
stalks, finely chopped 2 tomatoes, cubed

Directions:

In a bowl, combine the fennel with the chives, lime juice
and the other ingredients, toss well, divide into smaller
bowls and serve as an appetizer.

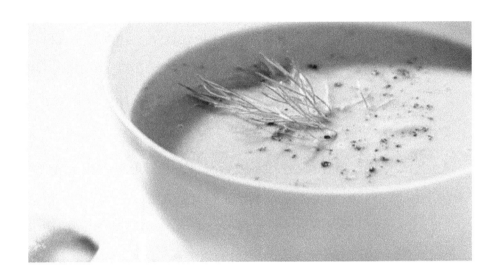

Chocolate Avocado Ice Cream

Preparation time: 1 hour and 10 minutes Cooking time: 0 minute Servings: 2

Ingredients:

4.5 ounces avocado, peeled, pitted 1/2 cup cocoa powder, unsweetened 1 tablespoon vanilla extract, unsweetened 1/2 cup and 2 tablespoons maple syrup 13.5 ounces coconut milk, unsweetened 1/2 cup water

Directions:

Add avocado in a food processor along with milk and then pulse for 2 minutes until smooth. Add remaining ingredients, blend until mixed, and then tip the pudding in a freezer-proof container. Place the container in a freezer and chill for freeze for 4 hours until firm, whisking every 20 minutes after 1 hour. Serve straight away.

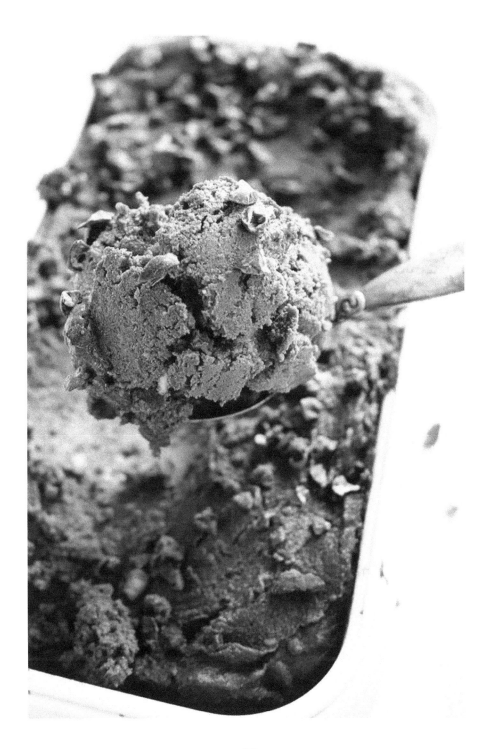

Mango Coconut Chia Pudding

Preparation time: 2 hours and 5 minutes Cooking time: 0 minute Servings: 1

Ingredients:

1 medium mango, peeled, cubed 1/4 cup chia seeds 2 tablespoons coconut flakes 1 cup coconut milk, unsweetened 1 1/2 teaspoons maple syrup

Directions:

Take a bowl, place chia seeds in it, whisk in milk until combined, and then stir in maple syrup. Cover the bowl with a plastic wrap; it should touch the pudding mixture and refrigerate for 2 hours until the pudding has set. Then puree mango until smooth, top it evenly over pudding, sprinkle with coconut flakes and serve.

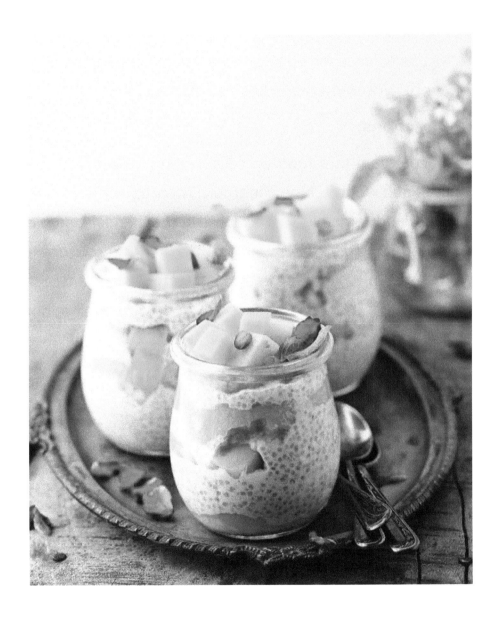

Strawberry Coconut Ice Cream

Preparation time: 5 minutes Cooking time: 0 minute Servings: 4

Ingredients:

4 cups frouncesen strawberries 1 vanilla bean, seeded 28 ounces coconut cream 1/2 cup maple syrup

Directions:

Place cream in a food processor and pulse for 1 minute until soft peaks come together. Then tip the cream in a bowl, add remaining ingredients in the blender and blend until thick mixture comes together. Add the mixture into the cream, fold until combined, and then transfer ice cream into a freezer-safe bowl and freeze for 4 hours until firm, whisking every 20 minutes after 1 hour. Serve straight away

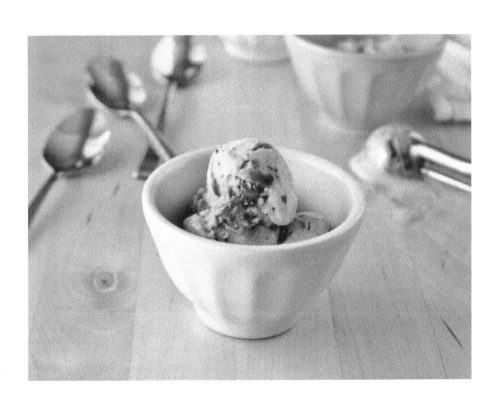

Chocolate Peanut Butter Energy Bites

Preparation time: 1 hour and 5 minutes Cooking time: 0 minute Servings: 4

Ingredients:

1/2 cup oats, old-fashioned 1/3 cup cocoa powder, unsweetened 1 cup dates, chopped 1/2 cup shredded coconut flakes, unsweetened 1/2 cup peanut butter

Directions:

Place oats in a food processor along with dates and pulse for 1 minute until the paste starts to come together. Then add remaining ingredients, and blend until incorporated and very thick mixture comes together. Shape the mixture into balls, refrigerate for 1 hour until set and then serve.

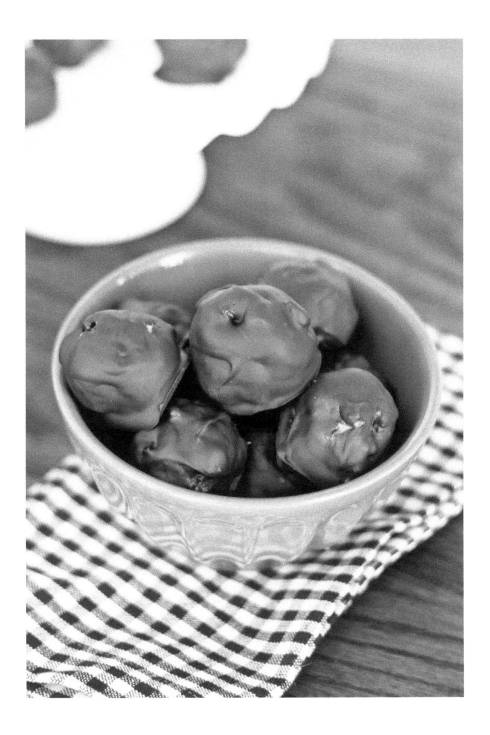

Rainbow Fruit Salad

Preparation time: 10 minutes Cooking time: 0 minute
Servings: 4

Ingredients:

For the Fruit Salad: 1 pound strawberries, hulled, sliced 1 cup kiwis, halved, cubed 1 1/4 cups blueberries 1 1/3 cups blackberries 1 cup pineapple chunks

For the Maple Lime Dressing: 2 teaspoons lime zest 1/4 cup maple syrup 1 tablespoon lime juice

Directions:

Prepare the salad, and for this, take a bowl, place all its ingredients and toss until mixed. Prepare the dressing, and for this, take a small bowl, place all its ingredients and whisk well. Drizzle the dressing over salad, toss until coated and serve.

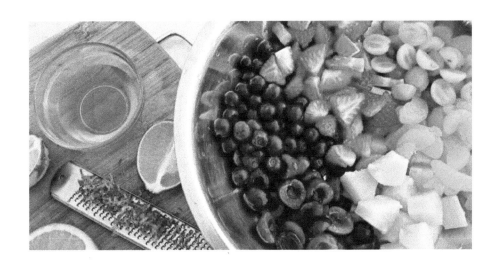

Dark Chocolate Bars

Preparation time:1 hour and10 minutes Cooking time:2 minutesServings: 12

Ingredients:

1 cup cocoa powder, unsweetened 3 Tablespoons cacao nibs 1/8 teaspoon sea salt 2 Tablespoons maple syrup 1 1/4 cup chopped cocoa butter 1/2 teaspoons vanilla extract, unsweetened 2 Tablespoons coconut oil

Directions:

Take a heatproof bowl, add butter, oil, stir, and microwave for 90 to 120 seconds until melts, stirring every 30 seconds. Sift cocoa powder over melted butter mixture, whisk well until combined, and then stir in maple syrup, vanilla, and salt until mixed. Distribute the mixture evenly between twelve mini cupcake liners, top with cacao nibs, and freeze for 1 hour until set. Serve straight away

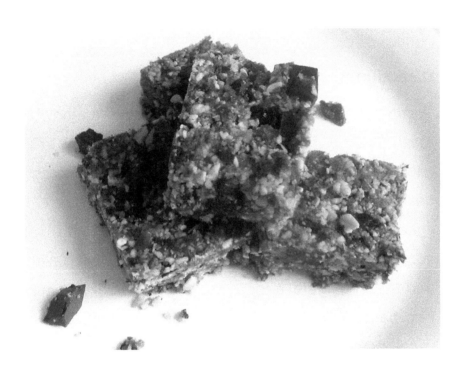

Chocolate and Avocado Truffles

Preparation time:1 hour and10 minutes Cooking time:1 minute Servings: 18

Ingredients:

1 medium avocado, ripe 2 tablespoons cocoa powder 10 ounces of dark chocolate chips

Directions:

Scoop out the flesh from avocado, place it in a bowl, then mash with a fork until smooth, and stir in 1/2 cup chocolate chips. Place remaining chocolate chips in a heatproof bowl and microwave for 1 minute until chocolate has melted, stirring halfway. Add melted chocolate into avocado mixture, stir well until blended, and then refrigerate for 1 hour. Then shape the mixture into balls, 1 tablespoon of mixture per ball, and roll in cocoa powder until covered. Serve straight away.

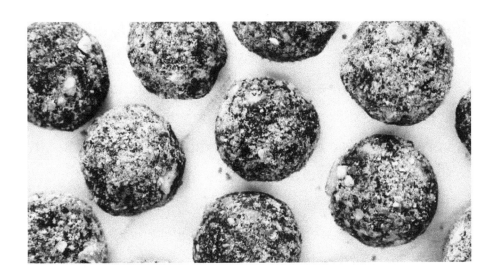

Peaches in Red Wine

Preparation time: 5 minutesCooking time: 40 minutes Servings: 2 **Ingredients:**

10 peaches 4½ cups red wine ¾ cup sugar 1 stick cinnamon, 2 inches long

Directions: Wash the peaches, handling them gently to avoid bruising. In a fairly large enameled saucepan, simmer the wine with the sugar and cinnamon until all the sugar is dissolved. Add the peaches and simmer them very gently for 8 minutes. Remove the saucepan from the heat and leave the peaches in the hot wine for about ½ hour. Spoon out the peaches, allow them to cool slightly, then carefully slip off their skins. Arrange them in an attractive serving dish, pour the wine over them, and chill for at least 1 hour.

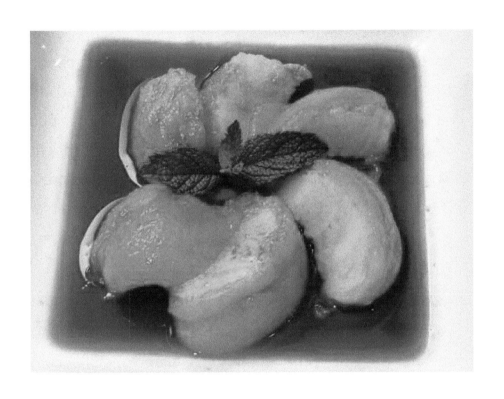

Garbanzo Croquettes

Preparation time: 5 minutesCooking time: 55 minutes
Servings: 2

Ingredients:

⅓ cup dried bulgur wheat ⅔ cup water 2 cups cooked garbanzo beans ¼ cup fresh lemon juice 3 Tbs. chopped fresh cilantro (coriander leaves) 1½ tsp. crushed dried red chilis ½ tsp. ground cumin 1 tsp. salt 3 Tbs. butter ⅛ tsp. cinnamon 1½ tsp. fresh-minced garlic 3 Tbs. flour ¾ cup hot vegetable broth 2 cups fine, dry bread crumbs 2 eggs, lightly beaten flour (about ⅔ cup) vegetable oil for deep frying

Directions: Soak the bulgur wheat in the water for 20 minutes, then drain it in a fine sieve, pressing out all the excess moisture. Mash the garbanzo beans with a potato masher and stir in the lemon juice, cilantro, chilis, cumin, and salt. Melt the butter in a small saucepan and add the cinnamon and garlic to it. Sauté for about 2 minutes, then stir in the 3 tablespoons flour. Cook the roux over low heat for several minutes, stirring often, then stir in the vegetable broth. Continue cooking and stirring the sauce until it is thick and smooth. Add it to the garbanzo bean mixture, along with the soaked bulgur and ½ of the breadcrumbs. Stir the mixture thoroughly, taste, and correct the seasoning if necessary. Chill the mixture for about 2 hours. Put the beaten eggs in a small, shallow bowl, the flour in another one, and the remaining 1 cup breadcrumbs in a third. Scoop up the croquette mixture by rounded tablespoonfuls and roll each one into a ball—they should be about the size of large walnuts. Roll each ball in flour until it is well coated. When all the balls have been floured, take one at a time and dip it first in the beaten eggs, then roll it quickly in the breadcrumbs until it is completely encrusted. Cook the croquettes in deep, hot vegetable oil, about 7 or 8 at a time, for 6 to 8 minutes, or until they are crisp and golden brown all over. Drain them on paper towels and keep them warm in the oven while cooking the rest. Serve.

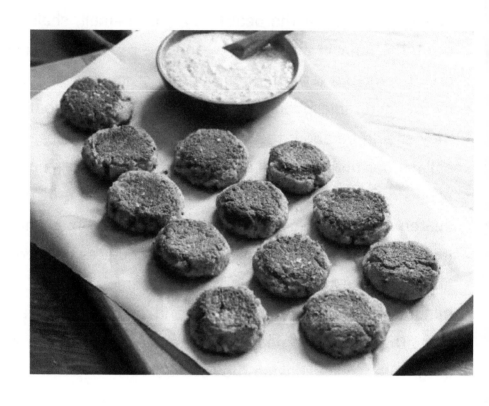

Apple & Spinach Juice

Preparation Time: 10 minutes Cooking Time: 0-minute
Servings: 2

Ingredients:

1½ cups spinach ½ grapefruit, sliced 2 apples, sliced 1 small ginger, sliced 2 stalks celery

Direction: Process the ingredients in your juicer following the order in the list. Pour juice into glasses and chill before serving.

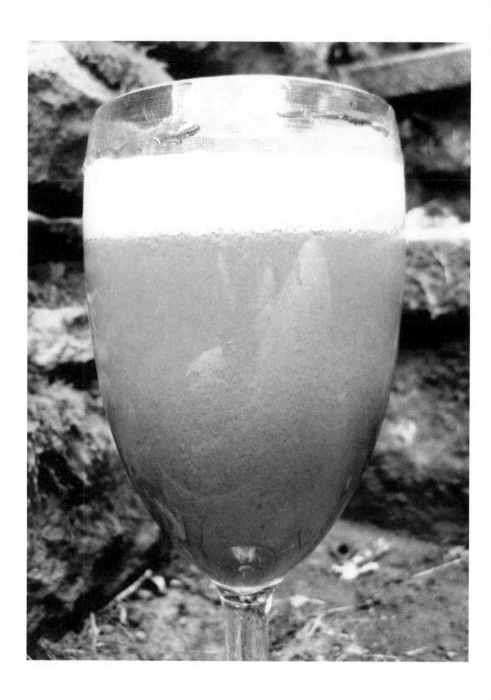

Fat Burger Bombs

Preparation time: 30 minutes Cooking time: 20 minutes Servings: 6

Ingredients:

12 slices uncured bacon, chopped 1 cup almond flour 2 eggs, beaten ½ pound ground beef What you'll need from the store cupboard: Salt and pepper to taste 3 tablespoons olive oil

Directions

In a mixing bowl, combine all ingredients except for the olive oil. Use your hands to form small balls with the mixture. Place in a baking sheet and allow it to set in the fridge for at least 2 hours. Once 2 hours is nearly up, preheat oven to 400oF. Place meatballs in a single layer in a baking sheet and brush the meatballs with olive oil on all sides. Cook for 20 minutes.

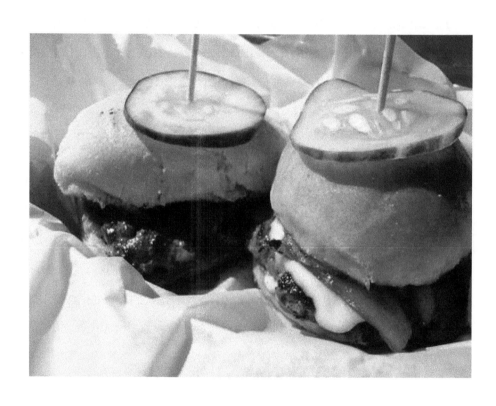

Lemon Ginger Bread

Preparation time: 15 minutes Cooking time: 35 minutes
1 loaf of bread.

Ingredients:

1 ¾ cup whole wheat flour ½ cup sugar 1 tsp. cinnamon 1 tsp. baking soda ½ tsp. nutmeg ½ tsp. salt ½ tsp. cloves 2 tbsp. grated ginger zest from two lemons 1 tbsp. olive oil 1 cup water 2 tsp. apple cider vinegar For After Baking: 1 cup powdered sugar juice from two lemons

Directions:

Begin by preheating the oven to 350 degrees Fahrenheit. Next, mix together all of the dry ingredients. Afterwards, form two holes in the dry mixture. Pour the vinegar in one hole, and pour the oil in the other hole. Add the water, and then mix well. Next, pour the created batter into a bread loaf pan and bake the bread for thirty-five minutes. To the side, mix together the lemon juice and the powdered sugar. Pour this mixture over the top of the bread after it cools, and enjoy.

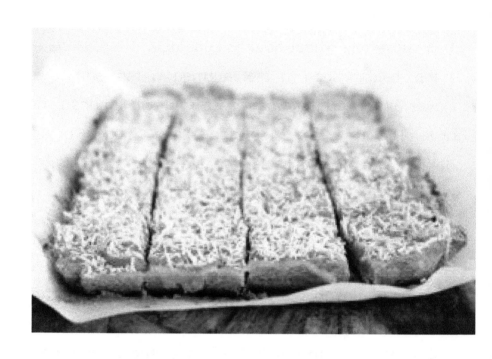

Vegetable Cheese Pizza

Preparation time: 15 minutes Cooking time: 25 minutes Servings: 5

Ingredients:

1 ¼ cups sharp provolone cheese, shredded 1 small red bell pepper, cut into pieces 4 garlic cloves, thinly sliced ¼ tsp salt 2 tbsp balsamic vinegar Vegetable cooking spray 1 small sweet onion 1 tsp olive oil 1 tbsp fresh or dried thyme leaves 10 oz can refrigerated pizza vegan-crust dough

Directions:

Set the oven at 425 degrees. Coat the baking sheet with cooking spray. Unroll the pizza dough in the baking sheet. Fold it under the edges to form a circle. Bake for 7 minutes at 425 degrees. Increase heat to 500 degrees. Combine thyme, olive oil, red bell pepper, balsamic vinegar, salt, garlic and red bell pepper. Toss the mixture in a bowl. Spread it in the baking sheet. Bake for 15 minutes at 500 degrees. Stir the mixture halfway through cooking. Reduce the temperature to 425 degrees. Spread half of the cheese mixture on top of the pizza crust. Arrange the roasted vegetables on top of cheese. Top with the remaining cheese. Bake it for 425 degrees at 12 minutes until crust is browned.

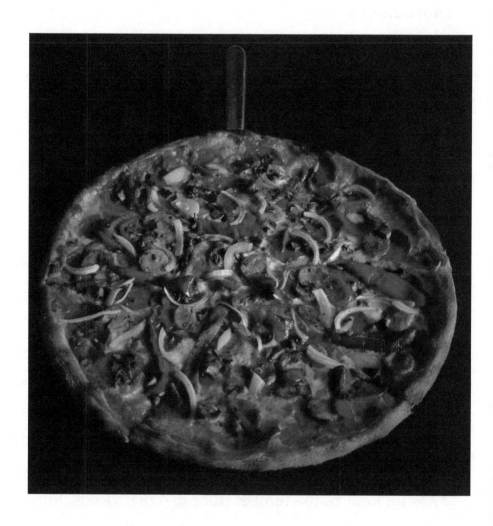

Potato nuggets

Preparation time: 10 minutes | Cooking time: 30 minutes | Servings: 4

Ingredients:

2 boiled potatoes 3 tbsp. cheddar cheese ½ tsp ginger ½ tsp herbs ½ tsp chili ¼ tsp pepper Salt as per taste 2 tbsp. coriander leaves ¼ cup bread crumbs

For coating:

1 cup bread crumbs ¼ tsp pepper ¼ tsp salt ¼ cup of water Oil ¼ cup cornflour

Directions:

Take a bowl, add boiled potatoes, cheddar cheese, ginger, garlic, pepper, chili, salt, coriander and herbs. Mix all the Ingredients well until well combined. Now add the bread crumbs and mix. It helps to join the potato balls together. Now in another bowl, prepare the material for coating. Take a small bowl, add cornflour, pepper, salt and water mix them and prepare a thick batter. In a small bowl, pour the bread crumbs separately for coating. Now take a small portion of potato mixture and make balls or any shape of your choice. Roll them into corn flour batter then in bread crumbs. Repeat the process until all done.

In a pan, heat the oil for frying and fry the prepared potatoes in it. Serve the hot nuggets with sauce.

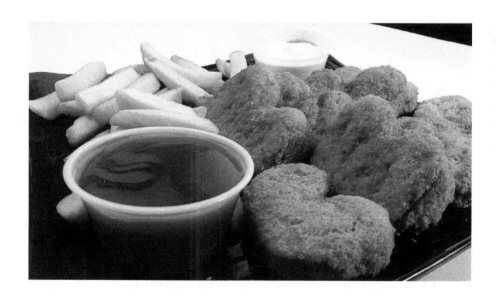

Teriyaki veggie crunch rolls

Preparation time: 25 minutes | Cooking time: 50 minutes | Servings: 3-4 rolls

Ingredients:

For rice: 1 cup of brown rice 1 tbsp. can sugar 1 ½ tbsp. organic rice vinegar ¼ tsp sea salt

For filling: 1 small Japanese yam 1 carrot ½ avocado ½ cucumber 3-4 toasted nori sheets ¾ cup brown rice cereal ½ cup ginger pickled For the teriyaki sauce: ½ cup wheat-free tamari ½ cup can sugar 2 tsp brown rice vinegar 2 tsp ginger pickled ¼ tsp garlic powder 2 tbsp. pineapple juice 2 tsp arrowroot powder 1 tbsp. water

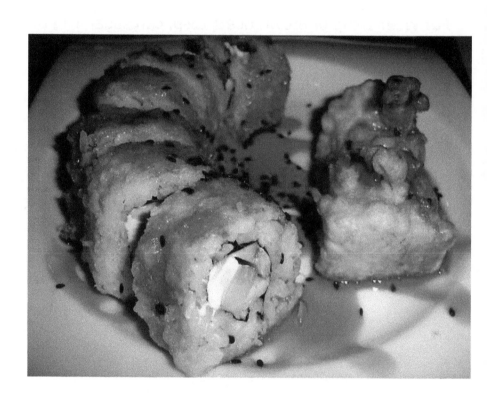

Potato pancake

Preparation time: 25 minutes | Cooking time: 25 minutes | Servings: 20

Ingredients:

2 potatoes ½ cup oat flour 1 large zucchini 1 tsp baking powder ½ yellow onion ½ tsp black pepper

Directions:

In a bowl, add potatoes and yellow onion and set aside. In another bowl, pour oat flour, baking powder and pepper to mix them well. Now add the vegetables into the flour mixture and combine them together. Preheat oven at 425 degrees. Set parchment paper in baking pan. Take potato mixture with the spoon and formed a round ball, then flatten with the hand and put in a baking pan. Prepare 20 cakes with equal size. Bake them for 12 minutes, then flip the side and bake again for another 12 to 13 minutes. Serve the crispy potato pancake with any sauce of your choice.

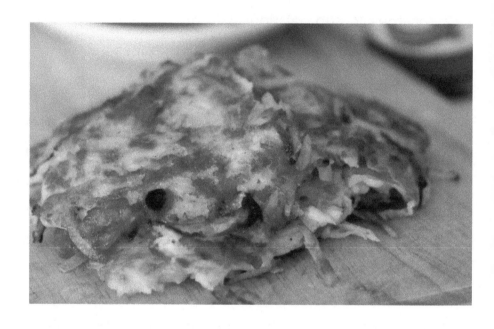

Herbed hummus

Preparation time: 20 minutes | Cooking time: 5 minutes | Servings: 8

Ingredients:

1 cup basil leaves 1 cup of vegetable broth ½ cup tarragon leaves ½ cup fresh parsley leaves 4 cups cooked beans 1 lemon juice 2 tbsp. sesame seeds 2 garlic cloves ¼ cup chopped chives

Directions:

Clean the basil leaves and let them dry. Take a food processor and add basil leaves, beans, vegetable broth, parsley leaves, lemon juice, sesame seeds and garlic. Blend the Ingredients well until smooth and thick in density. Stir in the chives and put in the refrigerator for 20 minutes. You can store the hummus for 4 days in the refrigerator.

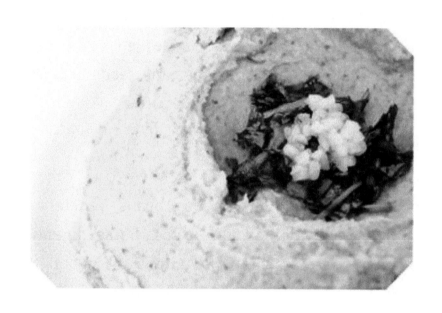

Cajun Spiced Pecans

Preparation time: 5 minutes Cooking time: 10 minutes Servings: 12

Ingredients:

1-pound pecan halves ¼ cup melted butter 1 packet Cajun seasoning mix ¼ teaspoon ground cayenne pepper What you'll need from the store cupboard: Salt and pepper to taste

Directions

Preheat oven to 400oF. In a small bowl, whisk well-melted butter, Cajun seasoning, cayenne, salt, and pepper. Place pecan halves on a cookie sheet. Drizzle with sauce. Toss well to coat. Pop in the oven and roast for 10 minutes. Let it cool completely, serve, and enjoy.

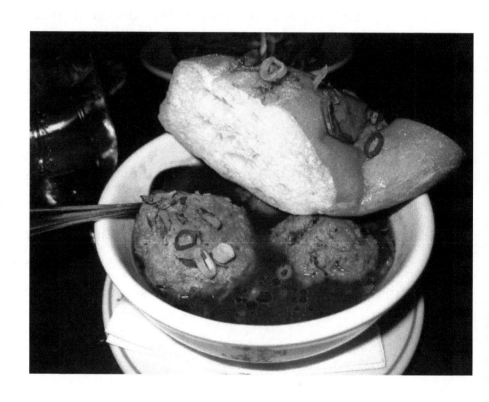

Garden Salad Wraps

Preparation Time: 15 minutes cooking time: 10 minutes serves: 4 wraps

Ingredients

6 tablespoons olive oil 1 pound extra-firm tofu, drained, patted dry, and cut into 1/2-inch strips 1 tablespoon soy sauce 1/4 cup apple cider vinegar 1 teaspoon yellow or spicy brown mustard 1/2 teaspoon salt 1/4 teaspoon freshly ground black pepper 3 cups shredded romaine lettuce 3 ripe Roma tomatoes, finely chopped 1 large carrot, shredded 1 medium English cucumber, peeled and chopped 1/3 cup minced red onion 1/4 cup sliced pitted green olives 4 (10-inch) whole-grain flour tortillas or lavash flatbread

Directions

In a large skillet, heat 2 tablespoons of the oil over medium heat. Add the tofu and cook until golden brown, about 10 minutes. Sprinkle with soy sauce and set aside to cool. In a small bowl, combine the vinegar, mustard, salt, and pepper with the remaining 4 tablespoons oil, stirring to blend well. Set aside. In a large bowl, combine the lettuce, tomatoes, carrot, cucumber, onion, and olives. Pour on the dressing and toss to coat. To assemble wraps, place 1 tortilla on a work surface and spread with about one-quarter of the salad. Place a few strips of tofu on the tortilla and roll up tightly. Slice in half 76.

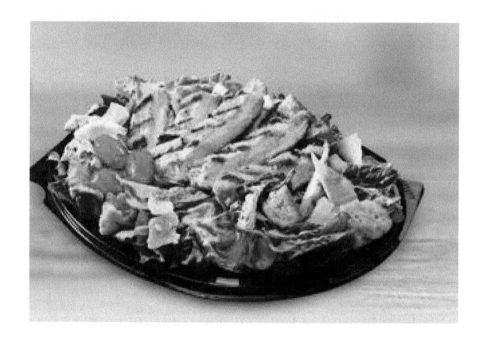

Tamari Toasted Almonds

Preparation Time: 2 minutes cooking time: 8 minutes serves: ½ cup

Ingredients

½ cup raw almonds, or sunflower seeds 2 tablespoons tamari, or soy sauce 1 teaspoon toasted sesame oil

Directions

Preparing the Ingredients. Heat a dry skillet to medium-high heat, then add the almonds, stirring very frequently to keep them from burning. Once the almonds are toasted, 7 to 8 minutes for almonds, or 3 to 4 minutes for sunflower seeds, pour the tamari and sesame oil into the hot skillet and stir to coat. You can turn off the heat, and as the almonds cool the tamari mixture will stick to and dry on the nuts.

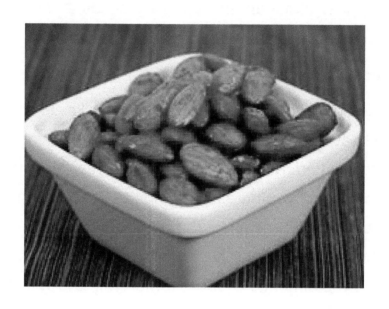

Kale Chips

Preparation Time: 5 minutes cooking time: 25 minutes serves: 2

Ingredients

1 large bunch kale 1 tablespoon extra-virgin olive oil ½ teaspoon chipotle powder ½ teaspoon smoked paprika ¼ teaspoon salt

Directions

Preparing the Ingredients. Preheat the oven to 275ºF. Line a large baking sheet with parchment paper. In a large bowl, stem the kale and tear it into bite-size pieces. Add the olive oil, chipotle powder, smoked paprika, and salt. Toss the kale with tongs or your hands, coating each piece well. Spread the kale over the parchment paper in a single layer. Bake for 25 minutes, turning halfway through, until crisp. Cool for 10 to 15 minutes before dividing and storing in 2 airtight containers.

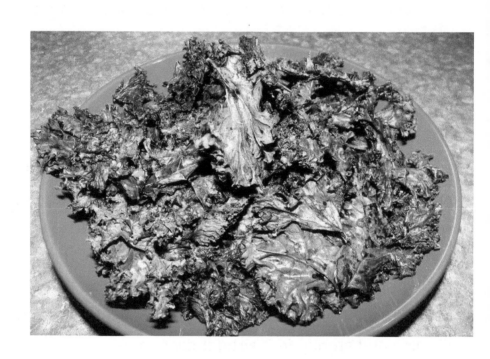

Savory Seed Crackers

Preparation Time: 5 minutes cooking time: 50 minutes serves: 20 crackers

Ingredients

¾ cup pumpkin seeds (pepitas) ½ cup sunflower seeds ½ cup sesame seeds ¼ cup chia seeds 1 teaspoon minced garlic (about 1 clove) 1 teaspoon tamari or soy sauce 1 teaspoon vegan Worcestershire sauce ½ teaspoon ground cayenne pepper ½ teaspoon dried oregano ½ cup water

Directions

Preparing the Ingredients. Preheat the oven to 325ºF. Line a rimmed baking sheet with parchment paper. In a large bowl, combine the pumpkin seeds, sunflower seeds, sesame seeds, chia seeds, garlic, tamari, Worcestershire sauce, cayenne, oregano, and water. Transfer to the prepared baking sheet, spreading out to all sides. Bake for 25 minutes. Remove the pan from the oven, and flip the seed "dough" over so the wet side is up. Bake for another 20 to 25 minutes, until the sides are browned. Cool completely before breaking up into 20 pieces. Divide evenly among 4 glass jars and close tightly with lids.

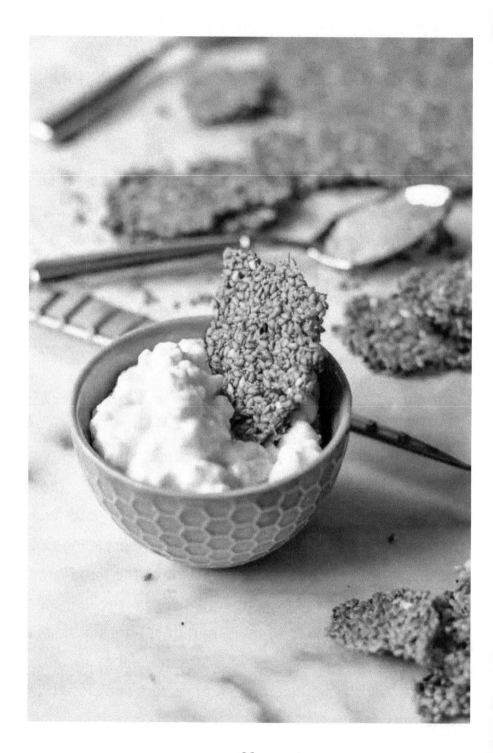

Refried Bean and Salsa Quesadillas

Preparation Time: 5 minutes cooking time: 6 minutes serves: 4 quesadillas

Ingredients

1 tablespoon canola oil, plus more for frying 11/2 cups cooked or 1 (15.5-ounce) can pinto beans, drained and mashed 1 teaspoon chili powder 4 (10-inch) whole-wheat flour tortillas 1 cup tomato salsa, homemade or store-bought 1/2 cup minced red onion (optional)

Directions

In a medium saucepan, heat the oil over medium heat. Add the mashed beans and chili powder and cook, stirring, until hot, about 5 minutes. Set aside. To assemble, place 1 tortilla on a work surface and spoon about 1/4 cup of the beans across the bottom half. Top the beans with the salsa and onion, if using. Fold top half of the tortilla over the filling and press slightly. In large skillet heat a thin layer of oil over medium heat. Place folded quesadillas, 1 or 2 at a time, into the hot skillet and heat until hot, turning once, about 1 minute per side. Cut quesadillas into 3 or 4 wedges and arrange on plates. Serve immediately.

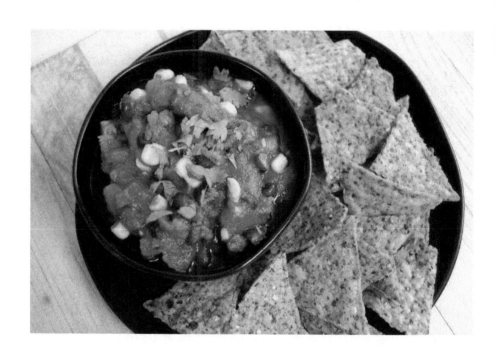

Garlic Dip

Preparation time: 10 minutes Cooking time: 0 minutes
Servings: 6

Ingredients:

1 cup coconut cream 4 garlic cloves, minced 2
tablespoons parsley, chopped 1 tablespoon lemon juice
Salt and black pepper to the taste 1 teaspoon garlic
powder 1 tablespoon cilantro, chopped

Directions:

In a blender, combine the cream with the garlic, parsley
and the other ingredients, pulse well, divide into small
bowls and serve as a party dip.

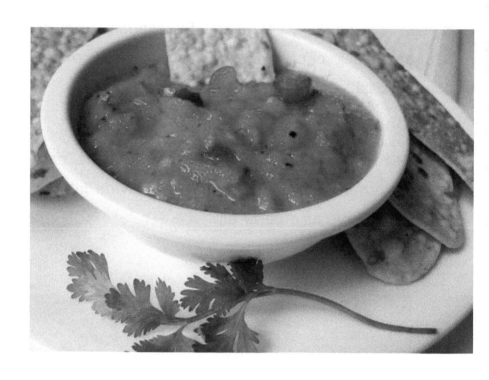

Coconut Spinach Balls

Preparation time: 10 minutes Cooking time: 0 minutes Servings: 12

Ingredients:

1 cup coconut cream 2 cups spinach, chopped 1 cup coconut, unsweetened and shredded 1 tablespoon psyllium powder 2 cups cashew cheese, grated 2 tablespoons Italian seasoning Salt and black pepper to the taste 1 teaspoon parsley, dried

Directions:

In a bowl, mix the spinach with the cream and the other ingredients except the coconut and stir well. Shape medium balls out of this mix, dredge them in coconut, arrange on a platter and serve.

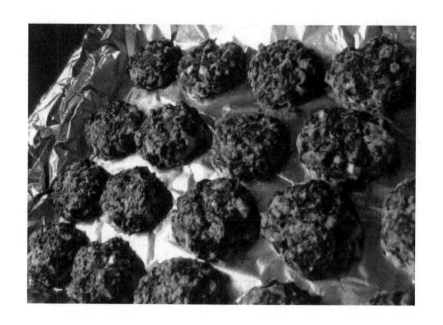

Veggie Snack

Preparation time: 5 minutes Cooking time: 20 minutes Servings: 4

Ingredients:

1 cup cherry tomatoes, halved 1 cup radish, halved 1 cup black olives, pitted 2 tablespoons olive oil 1 teaspoon chili powder Salt and black pepper to the taste ½ teaspoon Italian seasoning A pinch of red pepper flakes, crushed 1 teaspoon garlic powder

Directions:

In a bowl, combine the tomatoes with the radishes and the other ingredients, toss, spread the veggies on a baking sheet lined with parchment paper and bake at 420 degrees F for 20 minutes. Divide the veggies into bowls and serve as a snack.

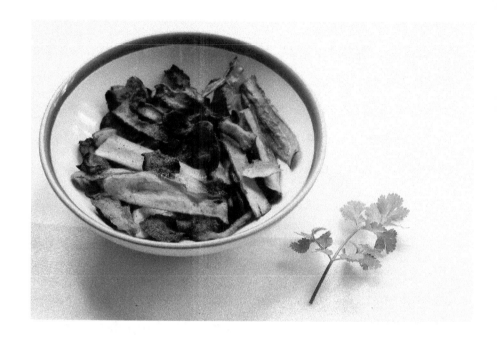

Pleasant Lemonade

Servings: 10 servings Preparation time: 3 hours and 15 minutes

Ingredients:

Cinnamon sticks for serving 2 cups of coconut sugar 1/4 cup of honey 3 cups of lemon juice. fresh 32 fluid ounce of water

Directions:

Using a 4-quarts slow cooker, place all the ingredients except for the cinnamon sticks and stir properly. Cover it with the lid, then plug in the slow cooker and cook it for 3 hours on the low heat setting or until it is heated thoroughly. When done, stir properly and serve with the cinnamon sticks

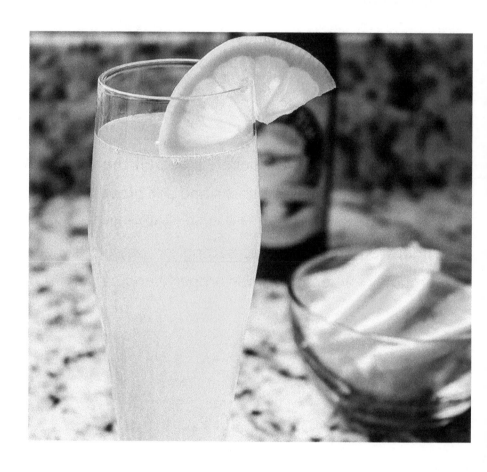

Vegetable & Tomato Juice

Preparation Time: 10 minutes Cooking Time: 0 minute
Servings: 2

Ingredients:

1 cup Romaine lettuce ¼ cup fresh chives, chopped 2 tomatoes, sliced 1 red bell pepper, sliced 2 stalks celery, chopped 1 carrot, chopped

Direction:

Process the ingredients in proper order using a juicer. Pour the juice into glasses and serve.

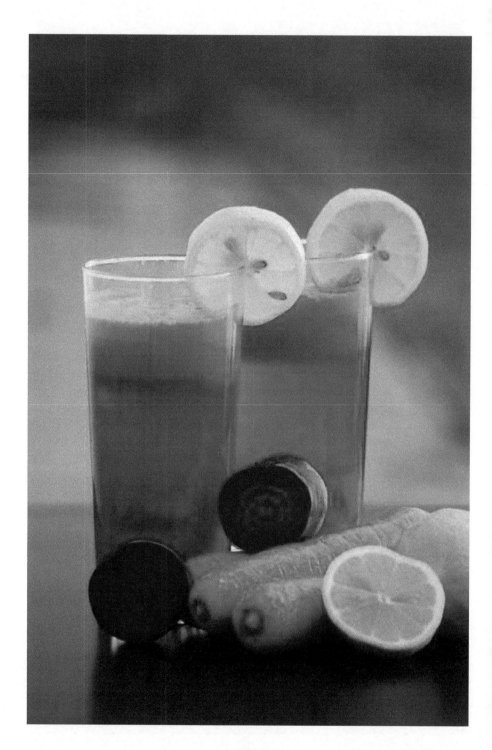

Easy Baked Parmesan Chips

Preparation time: 5 minutesCooking time: 10 minutes
Servings: 10

Ingredients:

1 cup grated Parmesan cheese, low fat 1 tablespoon olive oil What you'll need from the store cupboard: none

Directions

Lightly grease a cookie sheet and preheat oven to 400°F. Evenly sprinkle parmesan cheese on a cookie sheet into 10 circles. Place them about ½-inch apart. Drizzle with oil Bake until lightly browned and crisped. Let it cool, evenly divide into suggested servings and enjoy.

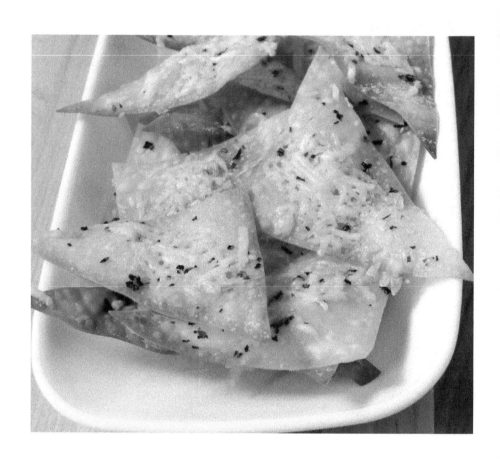

Lightning Source UK Ltd.
Milton Keynes UK
UKHW020810250521
384334UK00001B/69